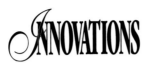

Opportunities for
Daily Choice Making

Linda M. Bambara

Freya Koger

Diane Browder
Editor, *Innovations*

American Association on Mental Retardation

Printed in the United States of America.

Published by
American Association on Mental Retardation
444 North Capitol Street, NW
Suite 846
Washington, DC 20001-1512

The points of view expressed herein are those of the authors and do not necessarily represent the official policy or opinion of the American Association on Mental Retardation. Publication does not imply endorsement by the editor, the association, or its individual members.

Library of Congress Cataloging-in-Publication Data
Bambara, Linda M., 1952–
      Opportunities for daily choice making/Linda M. Bambara, Freya Koger.
          p. cm. — (Innovations, ISSN 1072-4036; no. 8)
      Includes bibliographical references.
      ISBN 0-940898-44-6
      1. Developmentally disabled—Counseling of. 2. Choice (Psychology)
I. Koger, Freya, 1963-. II. Title. III. Series: Innovations (Washington, D.C.: 1994);
no. 8.
HV1570.835 1996
362.1'968—dc20   96-35425
                                                       CIP

Table of Contents

Introduction

Not providing opportunities for choice making may be viewed as a form of discrimination against people with disabilities.

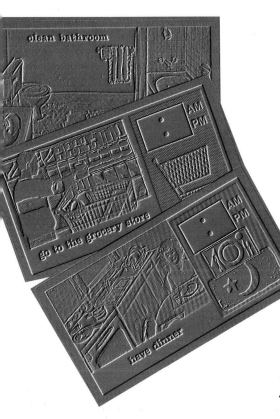

Imagine Your Life Without Choices

Imagine that you are dependent upon another to help you navigate through life's daily activities. Imagine further that this guide makes all decisions for you. Imagine starting your day being told when to wake up, what to wear, and what to eat. You are particularly hungry this morning. You head for the kitchen, but you hear, "No, no, no, shower first!" You want to wear your comfortable jeans, but dress trousers are more befitting of your age. You reach for the cold cereal, but hot oatmeal is more nutritiously sound, besides cold cereals are reserved for Saturdays only. There are even rules for brushing your teeth. You wet your toothbrush after you apply the toothpaste, not before.

You arrive at work. Great, the morning newspaper is on your desk. *I wonder who won last night,* you think, but before you have a chance to touch the paper, your guide removes it from your reach. "Newspapers are for breaks," you are reminded. "Work first, then break." You know better than to request a cup of coffee; coffee is also reserved for breaks. Your guide hands you your daily assignments. *Not a bad load,* you think, *but please, give me anything but that horrible assignment first.* You are promptly handed the dreaded assignment. Your guide pats you on your back. "You work so much better when you get those difficult jobs out of the way."

Lunch time. *Let me see,* you say to yourself. *Today is Wednesday, so it must be turkey.* You

1

open your sandwich bag, and of course you are right. You don't mind turkey sandwiches, but this predictability is so boring. Even jelly on a Wednesday would be more exciting.

The day drags on. It's about four o'clock, mid-August, and hot. You head home, weary. You feel your body collapsing as you open the door. "Boy, do we have a busy schedule planned for you this evening!" your guide enthusiastically says. "Remember? We scheduled to clean your closet today! And then, because you worked so hard, we'll go bowling right after dinner. I know how much you love bowling!"

For the first time today, you resist. "I want, I need a nap now," you protest, "and I don't feel much like bowling."

"Now, now, now, once you get started it won't be so bad," your guide says. "Besides, chores first, then play!" You dig in your heels, only to find yourself being gently but firmly escorted to your closet door.

Somehow you manage to get through closet cleaning, dinner, and bowling. Finally you collapse on the couch. Sleep surrounds you immediately. Ah, peace. "Come on, wake up, you sleepy head," your guide says as she nudges you. "Beds are for sleeping, not couches. Besides, you haven't brushed your teeth yet. Come on let's go." And so it goes.

The Lives of People With Developmental Disabilities

It is difficult to imagine our lives without choices. Life without choice is a scenario few of us could or would tolerate. Indeed, many of us get testy just thinking about being told what to do. We make hundreds of choices each day. Choice is the primary vehicle through which we express preferences and direct the activities in our lives.

Although we may take choice making for granted, choice is a cherished component of everyday life.

Yet for people with developmental disabilities, opportunities for choice making are routinely absent. People who are most dependent upon others for support, due to the severity of their cognitive or physical limitations, are most vulnerable to having the least amount of choice and control in their lives. If choice making is valued, how did it come to pass that people with developmental disabilities are often denied such precious opportunities? We are unaware of any public declaration: "Thou shall not present choice to people with disabilities." And yet, often unknowingly, our attitudes and actions toward people with disabilities have created systemic barriers that have effectively preempted opportunities for choice.

Barriers to Choice Making

People with disabilities, including adolescents and adults, are often viewed as perpetual children who need to be protected. Opportunities for choice making are often overlooked. Teachers, parents, and support staff often fall into caregiving roles, because of intense physical and cognitive limitations. While most caregivers have the individual's best interests at heart, daily routines are built frequently around the caregiver's organizational needs and not necessarily the individual's preferences.

Professional training has also preempted opportunities for choice. Until recently, training programs failed to discuss the importance of choice making or even how to teach choice making to people who have limited expressive skills. As a result, educational goals even for adults are often selected without learner input. Instructors are guided to decide what to teach, how to teach, and even when to teach. Further, ıce instruction is planned, teachers are held ccountable to their goals. "I have to teach this; it in my student's IEP (or IHP or IPP or . . .)!" :ofessionals may fear that if they deviate from eir instructional plans, supervisors may think ey are not doing their jobs. Unfortunately, rigid lherence to instructional plans developed ıthout learner involvement leaves little room for exibility, student control, or choice making.

Not providing opportunities for choice aking may be viewed as a form of discrimina- ɔn against people with disabilities. For people ıthout disabilities, choice opportunities are radually increased from childhood and adoles- ɛnce until as adults they take on full autonomy ıd control. Because of the attitudinal and system- ic barriers to choice, people with developmental sabilities are denied this important opportunity to ıve control in their lives. While it may be argued at some people with disabilities do not have the kills for choice making or may make poor ecisions, which are not in their best interests or ɛ incompatible with their educational or ıbilitation goals, the question becomes, "How ɔes anyone learn responsible choice making ıthout the opportunity to make choices?" This ɔlds true for all of us.

Why Is Choice Making Important?

'e need only look at our own lives to understand hy choice is important. There are several ɛasons. First, *choice leads to personal satisfac- ɔn and quality of life.* Choice allows us to ıild our daily routines around preferences and ɪrect the activities that are important to us. All ɛople have the ability to choose at some level. he extent to which we can build our lives around ɪeferences, whether that means having a cup of ɔffee in the morning before showering or going

for a quiet walk in the evening, contributes directly to our happiness.

Second, *choice prepares learners for independence.* Independence is more than learning a set of tasks for daily living. True independence requires autonomy—being in control, being able to make decisions about what to do and when to do it. It requires that we weigh alternatives, make informed decisions, and learn from our mistakes. When people with disabilities are denied the opportunity to make choices, they are also denied the opportunity to learn these critical skills for independent living.

Third, *choice increases motivation to learn.* Creative teachers, parents, and employers have known this for years. Recent scientific data demonstrates that when people with disabilities are given the opportunity to choose among tasks, whether the tasks are school-, home-, or work-related, they participate longer and perform better than when tasks are assigned to them. For some people this holds true when the same tasks are involved. That is, some people may refuse to participate in an activity when told what to do. Yet they may happily engage in that very activity when given a choice between the refused activity and another. Why? Because being in control is in itself a motivator for participation. Choice making invites the individual to learn.

> Choice is primarily a quality-of-life variable. In addition, choice may result in many positive benefits for people with and without disabilities including increased participation in activities, better perfor- mance on tasks, and the prevention of problem behaviors.
>
> —**Bannerman, Sheldon, Sherman, & Harchik (1990)**

Fourth, *choice may prevent problem behaviors.* Behavioral excesses, such as repeated refusals, tantrums, and aggression, are often a result of the lack of choice and control. Problem behaviors may be forms of protests that occur when people are told what to do or are forced to engage in disliked activities. A common reaction to such protests is to tighten control (e.g., "You're not going to get away with that!") and provide even less choice. Sadly, this only exacerbates the problem, leading to a downward cycle—less and less choice causing increasingly more problem behaviors.

While some people with developmental disabilities express their frustrations aggressively, others give up. When people learn that they have no influence over others because they have no choices or because their protests are consistently ignored, they become sullen and withdrawn. This phenomenon, called *learned helplessness,* is just as severe a problem as behavioral excesses. The individual loses all motivation for learning and becomes totally dependent on others for direction. Fortunately, problem behaviors caused by the absence of choice and control can be reversed. Research demonstrates that when people with disabilities are provided with choices, problem behaviors decrease and participation in activities increases.

The Concept of Shared Control

Choice making does not mean having the freedom to choose independent from all constraints. We raise this issue because choice making can be conceptualized to the extreme. When misunderstood, it can inappropriately be used as an excuse not to provide choice or appropriate supports to people with developmental disabilities. One example is allowing an individual to jump out of a

> Choice making does not mean the freedom to do whatever one wants. It is a process of shared control.
>
> —**Carr & Colleagues (1994)**

second story window, because that is what the individual chooses to do. Of course this is a ridiculous concept.

Choice making does not involve the freedom to do whatever one wants. Choice making is a process of shared control, negotiated within the boundaries of constraints. The challenge is to ensure that the constraints are those that are imposed by society and are not arbitrarily so narrow as to discriminate against people with disabilities. For example, one commonly held standard is that we have more freedom at home than at work to make choices. Once we choose where we want to work, we must abide by the rules set up by our employer. Choices are made within those constraints. By contrast, at home we have considerably more latitude in choosing what to do, but even there our freedom is curtailed by the people with whom we share our home. Chores, for example, are negotiated among family members and roommates, and we are asked to respect the property and privacy of others.

Concerns about health and safety are other acceptable constraints. Few of us have qualms about setting firm limits for loved ones who engage in self-hurting behaviors such as poor dietary habits or drug or alcohol abuse. It is the same for people with developmental disabilities. Walking alone in a busy downtown area is not an acceptable choice if the person has not yet learned how to cross streets safely.

Constraints are also imposed by one's age and culture. We generally accept that children ave tighter limitations imposed on them than adults, but teachers and parents know that even within relatively tight boundaries children need to feel as if they are in control if learning is to be successful. The boundaries of choice for children are influenced by culture. Some cultures expect children to make greater choices than typical in European-American traditions, whereas other cultures postpone many choices until adolescence.

When supporting people with developmental disabilities, recognize the concept of shared control. Guide people to recognize their limits even as they discover the multitude of options available within reasonably set boundaries. Further, as teachers, parents, and support staff who work with people with disabilities, we must constantly evaluate ourselves to ensure that constraints are normalized and acceptable for people without disabilities of the same age and cultural background.

Purpose of This Book

The purpose of this book is to provide three strategies for increasing choice opportunities for people with developmental disabilities. Because choice opportunities are easily overlooked, these strategies provide systematic methods for ensuring that simple but important daily choices are made available. This book is intended for teachers, support staff, parents, and anyone else who cares about people with disabilities. Although this book may be relevant for people with many diverse needs, our focus will be on people with moderate to severe intellectual disabilities.

We begin in chapter 2 by describing basic principles of choice making, drawing some important implications for instruction. These principles set the foundation for the strategies introduced in chapters 3 to 5. In chapter 3 we present how to teach basic choice-making skills to the passive learner who has not yet realized that choice making can make things happen. In chapter 4 we expand on this strategy by describing how to build in multiple choice-making opportunities across the day and within daily routines. In chapter 5 we introduce self-scheduling as a method for helping people plan their days and make choices about what they want to do and when to do it. Finally, in chapter 6 we summarize important concepts by addressing some common questions and concerns about choice making for people with developmental disabilities. We hope you find this book useful.

C H A P T E R **P** T W O

Principles of Choice Making

Whether simple or complex, all choice-making opportunities follow the same basic process.

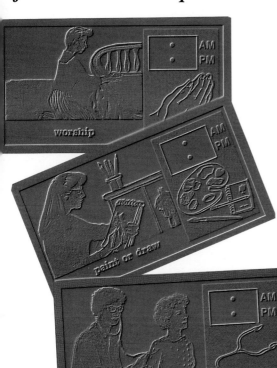

Understanding the Principles of Choice Making

There are many different types of choices, ranging from relatively simple ones, such as what cereal to eat or what bar of soap to wash with, to complex choices that require the individual to weigh the benefits of multiple alternatives, such as choosing where to live or how to spend money wisely. Opportunities for all types of choices are important. Our focus will be on how to present opportunities for relatively simple choices throughout the day. Whether simple or complex, all choice-making opportunities follow the same basic process illustrated in Figure 1. Understanding this process is important for teaching choice making as well as expanding choice opportunities throughout the day.

Choice Outcomes

Choice is simply the act of selecting between two or more options. More important, choice results in two critical outcomes: expressions of preference and control. Preference is what the person likes relative to other options. We all have preferences. Choice allows us to clearly communicate our preference.

An observer may note someone's preference by observing the number of times the person chooses one option over another. For example, if an individual chooses strawberry ice cream more often than chocolate, we can assume that strawberry is preferred. But because preference is relative to the specific options made available, it

7

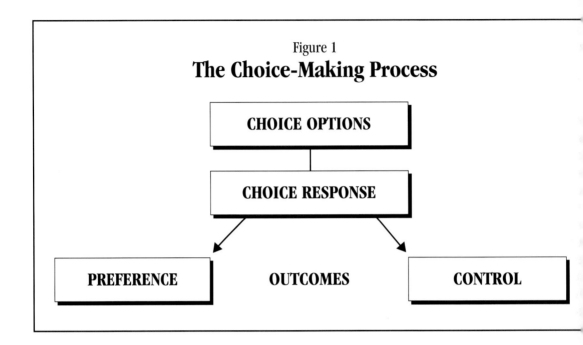

Figure 1
The Choice-Making Process

CHOICE OPTIONS

CHOICE RESPONSE

PREFERENCE   OUTCOMES   CONTROL

is continually changing. For example, presented with all possible ice cream flavors, strawberry may be most preferred. However, when presented a choice between chocolate and vanilla, the individual may choose chocolate even though this option is less preferred than strawberry. When an individual chooses options with equal frequency, sometimes choosing chocolate and sometimes choosing vanilla, we may conclude that the individual has no particular preference for one over the other. Relative to each other, both may be equally preferred. Conversely, if the individual chooses neither option, we may assume that both options are nonpreferred or disliked.

Control, or the ability to direct activities or the action of others, is the second critical outcome of choice. Control is often overlooked as an important outcome. But sometimes having the opportunity to choose is the most preferred outcome! The actions of people motivated by control can be baffling, because their behavior seems to contradict their preferences. "I gave Sue strawberry ice cream, her favorite, but now she says she hates it and won't eat it!" Actually, it may not be the ice cream that Sue hates, but the fact that she was not offered a choice. By refusing the ice cream, Sue obtains control over the situation.

Preference and control are equally important outcomes; if choice making is to be meaningful, person needs to be given opportunities to achieve both.

Choice Responses

Providing opportunities for choice making is meaningless unless the individual knows how to communicate a selection. When presented with a

> Obtaining a preferred option is an important outcome of choice. For some people, control may be an equally important outcome.
>
> —Bambara, Ager, & Koger (1994)

noice, some people with developmental disabili-
es may not respond at all or may respond in a
eemingly random way. In cases such as these,
noice making may need to be taught.

Teaching choice making involves three
mportant goals. The first is to teach learners how
• clearly communicate their selection to others.
eople communicate their choice selections in a
ariety of ways, such as stating or verbalizing their
reference; signing or gesturing; pointing or
eaching for a desired option; or looking at what
iey want. The second is to teach learners that
ieir selection will result in a preferred outcome.
earners need to understand that their choices
an impact their environment. The third goal is to
ive learners even greater control by teaching
iore sophisticated choice-making skills and
xpanding choice opportunities.

hoice Options

he type of choice *options* made available will
ifluence the individual's selection, even the
ecision to choose at all. Options must be
ieaningful. They must be presented in a way that
 understood and that results in outcomes that
re *important to the individual.* This means the
idividual must have sufficient experience with a
ariety of foods, objects, and activities to make
iformed selections. For example, presenting a
hoice between veal parmesan or beef stroganoff
 meaningless if the person has never tried either
ne. A "meaningful choice" also involves giving
ie individual what is selected—
r the individual will soon learn that his or her
election is not a viable option.

Implications for Presenting Choice Opportunities

From the preceding basic principles of choice
making we draw four implications for instruction.
These implications apply to all choice-making
strategies described in chapters 3, 4, and 5.

1. Present choice opportunities within the
    context of rich, stimulating environments in
    which the individual has frequent opportuni-
    ties to experience new materials, activities,
    and events. Old favorites quickly become
    boring options without opportunities to
    experience new things. The greater the
    experiences, the greater the options for
    choice making.

2. Present meaningful choice options that lead
    to preferred events and/or control. Options
    must be sufficiently motivating to invite a
    choice response.

3. Honor choice selections. Respond quickly,
    especially when teaching beginning choice-
    making skills. It is better to delay presenting
    a choice opportunity than not to respond to
    an individual's request.

4. Keep choice making inviting. By definition,
    choice means the opportunity to make
    selections free from coercion. Choice should
    never be used to force people to do some-
    thing that they do not want to do. "Do it, or
    I'll make you do it!" is not a "choice oppor-
    tunity."

T THREE

Teaching Beginning Choice-Making Skills

Through choice making, learners will realize they have the power to influence their environments and gain access to preferred events.

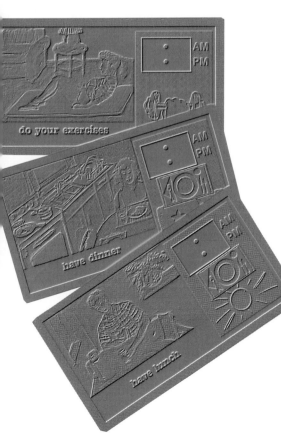

do your exercises

have dinner

have lunch

Learner Characteristics

Candidates for instruction in beginning choice-making skills are often described as passive learners. Although passive learners generally "cooperate" by participating in daily routines and activities, their participation is rarely active. Passive learners often fail to initiate activities on their own. They seem totally dependent on teachers, parents, or support staff for telling them what to do next. Once engaged in an activity, they make few, if any, spontaneous requests for materials or changes of activity. Although passive learners sometimes resist participation, resistance frequently takes the form of "doing nothing" as opposed to acting out, resulting in instructors prompting or "putting them through" the entire activity.

When presented with a choice opportunity, passive learners may appear apathetic. They do not respond with a choice selection, or they make nonmeaningful selections, such as always choosing the option on the right regardless of what option is presented.

There may be several reasons for the lack of choice making. Some learners may have never developed choice-making skills. Motor limitations can prevent some learners from making clear choice selections; others, who do not have physical limitations, may have never learned how

11

to communicate their choice selections. Still others may have learned how to signal choice but then stopped responding once they discovered that others are rarely responsive to their requests. Regardless of the reasons, choice making will need to be taught directly and systematically.

Overview of Teaching

The primary strategy for teaching beginning choice-making skills is (a) to prompt the learner to signal a choice made between liked options and (b) to provide the selected item upon each choice selection. Through repeated opportunities, the individual will learn how to make independent choice selections. More important, through choice making, learners will realize they have the power to influence their environments and gain access to preferred events.

We present instructional strategies for beginning choice-making skills in three components: (a) prepare for choice opportunities, (b) teach choice-making skills, and (c) evaluate success. Each component is described in detail.

Prepare for Choice Opportunities

Before teaching choice making, it is important to prepare how choice opportunities will be presented to the learner. This component involves four preparation steps as shown in Table 1.

Select Options Based on "Learner Likes"

The goal is to identify two or three pairs of items taken from several daily routines, such as mealtimes, leisure, or self-care activities, that the learner appears to enjoy. To maximize the number of choice opportunities presented in one routine, select options that can be presented in

---

Table 1

Component 1: Prepare for Choice Opportunities

1. **Select choice options based on "learner likes."**

   a. Select options from routine activities.

   b. Select items that can be presented in small portions or repeatedly introduced in turn-taking.

   c. Use real objects.

   d. Formulate two or three choice pairs.

2. **Identify and define a choice response.**
   Choose a response that:

   a. The learner can voluntarily control.

   b. Is easily performed.

   c. Is understood by others as a choice selection.

   d. Can be physically prompted if necessary.

3. **Choose routine activities (to present choice pairs).**

   a. Choose two or three routines, one for each choice pair.

   b. Choose routines where choices can be honored.

4. **Plan how to present choice opportunities.**

   a. Small-portion strategy.

   b. Turn-taking strategy.

small portions or that can be repeatedly introduced in a turn-taking fashion. Although choice
options may be presented verbally or through
symbols such as pictures, when teaching beginning choice-making skills, it is best to use actual
objects that can be given immediately. Examples
of appropriate choice options include favorite
foods or drinks, favorite activities that can be
represented by objects, such as listening to music
or playing with toys, and favorite materials used
during routine activities, such as scented markers
for coloring or foam soap for washing.

In the absence of choice-making skills,
identifying learner likes for certain objects or
activities may be difficult. But all people have
preferences; you can discover what a learner
likes or dislikes by simply observing learner
reactions to everyday events. When presented with
a particular material/activity, does the learner
respond by approaching it or rejecting it? An
approach response, defined as any voluntary
movement toward an item, maintaining contact
with an item, smiling or grimacing, or engaging in
positive verbalizations, may signal learner
preference. Examples include opening one's
mouth for food, relaxing when one's hair is
brushed, reaching for an item, turning toward the
source of sound, or looking at an item for long
periods. Conversely, a dislike for certain materials
or activities may be identified by observing a
learner's rejection response—any voluntary
movement away from an item, resistance to an
activity, or negative verbalizations. Examples
include pushing or turning away from objects,
tightening body movements, and making angry
sounds. By observing a learner's approach or
rejection responses to routine objects and
activities over several days, you will be able to
identify options that are liked and options to
avoid. Parents or other family members who
know the learner intimately are often best able to

> Approach and rejection behaviors are
> valid, nonverbal indicators of what a
> person likes and dislikes.
>
> —Sigafoos & Dempsey (1992)

discern learner interests. So if you are a teacher,
try to select options with parental input.

Once you have identified liked options, you
are ready to form two or three choice pairs.
Choice pairs should consist of one option that
seems very much liked by the individual plus
another enjoyable option that is related to the
same routine or activity. Nail polish and body
lotion, for example, are choice options related to
the same activity (e.g., grooming). To make
choice making easier for the learner, options
within a pair should be as maximally different
(visually or textually) as possible. For example,
even though orange juice and orange soda may
both be enjoyed by a learner, they would not form
a good choice pair, because the learner may have
difficulty telling the two apart. Pairing orange
juice with a different-colored drink, such as milk,
or another food, such as green Jell-O, are better
choice pairs because the options are more
distinguishable.

Identify and Define a Choice Response

In the second step of preparing for choice
opportunities, you will *identify and define a
choice response*. Learners can be taught to signal
their choice selections through a variety of
means, but the best response is one that (a) the
learner can voluntarily control (is not reflexive),
(b) is easily performed, (c) is readily recogniz-
able to others as a choice selection, and (d)
could be physically prompted if necessary. Your

objective is to identify the most efficient choice signal that will result in an immediate outcome. Remember, you want to teach the power of choice making!

When identifying a choice response, look for behaviors that the learner can already perform. If the learner knows how to reach for desired objects, then reaching might be a good choice response to select. If the learner can verbally label objects, choose labeling as a response. If the learner does not have a suitable choice response in his or her repertoire, identify a predictable behavior that the learner can perform. Look at approach behaviors for clues. For example, if a learner moves toward objects as a way of communicating "I like this," consider teaching an extension of this body movement that could be understood as choice selection by others. In this case, pointing or reaching toward a desired option might be good choice responses.

Once you have identified a choice response, define the response by describing exactly how the learner will indicate her choice selection. Use this definition to ensure that you are consistently teaching the learner to use the same choice response across all choice opportunities. The following is an example of a choice definition: "When presented with two options, Jon will indicate his choice by touching one of the items."

Choose Routine Activities

In the third preparation step, you will *choose routine activities during which you can present the choice pairs.* For the most part, the types of activities chosen will be determined by the nature of the choice pairs. For example, food-related choice pairs should be presented during mealtimes, leisure-related options during play activities, and self-care choice options during self-care or grooming routines. Choose one routine or activity (setting) for each choice pair. Ideally,

routines (or contexts for training trials) should be spread out across the day and occur frequentl during the week (three to five times) to provide sufficient opportunities for practice. Be sure to select routines in which you can give the learner your undivided attention and in which choices can be honored. For example, because dinnertime may be notoriously hectic for many families, it may not be an ideal routine for teaching initial choice-making skills. A late morning snack routine might be better suited for this purpose.

Plan to Present Choice Opportunities

Finally, in the last preparation step you will *plan how to present choice opportunities.* In each routine, you will be presenting the same choice pair several times. Consider how to present multiple choice opportunities, while still maintaining the learner's interest. There are two approaches. The first approach is to present small portions of an option at a time (e.g., small sips of juice, small amounts of paint for an art activity), and when the item is used up, present an opportunity for choice. The second approach is a variation of turn-taking in which an activity, such as hair brushing, is started, then stopped. Before restarting the activity, a choice opportunity is presented. In both approaches, the learner is motivated to make a choice selection by choosing to continue with the same option or by choosing something different by selecting the alternative.

Summary

By the end of this preparation component, you should have (a) identified two or three choice pairs that are based on learner likes, (b) identified and defined a choice response that you will be teaching, (c) identified two or three routines in which to present the choice pairs, and (d)

lanned how to present each choice pair several
mes during each activity. You are now ready to
egin teaching choice making.

Teach Choice Making

1 this component, you will present several
:aching opportunities or "trials" for choice
1aking in each of the identified routines. Basi-
ally, you will give the learner a choice between
vo options and repeat this opportunity several
mes during the activity. Presenting these choice
pportunities and responding to the learner's
hoice selections will teach the learner how to
1ake choices. Use the same teaching steps for
ach choice opportunity presented. These steps
re summarized in Table 2.

The first step is actually a practice trial in
hich you give the learner the opportunity to
imple each option in the choice pair. Before
resenting a choice, encourage the learner to
imple each option one at a time. If you are using
od options, encourage the learner to taste each
ne. If the options involve an activity, then model
e activity, involving the learner as much as
ossible. For example, play a little bit of the
usic from the tape player or encourage the
arner to try the scented markers. Sampling
lows the learner to know first-hand what the
ptions are.

While sampling, take note of the learner's
:sponses. Look for approach or rejection
:haviors. Does the learner seem to enjoy one
ption more than the other? If so, on subsequent
pportunities, when an independent choice
election is not made, prompt the learner to
:lect this option. After sampling, you are ready to
:gin your first teaching opportunity. Begin by
aking an offer. Place or hold the two options,
ft to right, in front of the learner. Be sure that
e learner looks at each one; you may need to

Table 2

Component 2:
Teach Choice Making

1. **Sample options.**

   a. Provide an opportunity for the learner to experience each option.

   b. Note approach/rejection responses.

2. **Offer options.**

   a. Place options before the learner, left/right.

   b. Direct scanning or looking.

3. **Ask.**

   "Do you want this or this?" or, "Which one do you want?"

4. **Wait.**

   5 to 10 seconds for a choice response.

5. **Respond immediately** if an independent choice response occurs.

   a. Give choice, remove other option.

   b. Praise.

6. **Prompt the choice response** if an independent response does not occur.

7. **Repair** — if the learner refuses an option; take option away, never force.

8. **Repeat steps 2 to 7** for another choice opportunity.

   a. Continue as long as the learner appears receptive to another choice trial.

   b. Vary the position of the options, left or right, on each trial.

direct scanning (e.g., "Look at what I have here, and here!"). While offering, ask (e.g., "Do you want the juice or the Jell-O?" or, "Which one would you like?"). Wait 5 to 10 seconds for the learner to make an independent choice response as defined in the preparation component. If a choice is made, then respond immediately; give the chosen option, remove the other item, and praise (e.g., "Great, you told me what you wanted!").

If the learner does not respond or attempts to make a choice selection but fails, then *you may need to prompt* the choice response. Use a verbal (e.g., "Touch the one you want"), a model (e.g., "Do this," the instructor demonstrates the choice response), or a physical prompt (e.g., the instructor physically guides the learner's hands to touch an option). Choose one prompt that will result in the learner making a choice response every time as defined. Use the same prompt across all teaching opportunities. When prompting, guide the learner to select the option that she seems to like the best. Use approach behaviors as clues. Is the learner staring at one option? During sampling, did the learner smile more often with one option? If you cannot be sure which option the learner seems to enjoy more, then prompt either one. Once you prompt a choice response, respond as if the learner made an independent choice selection (e.g., give the selected item, remove the other option, and praise).

Be aware that beginners will sometimes make mistakes. If the learner rejects an option after making an independent or prompted choice selection, then repair the situation. Remove the unwanted item immediately. Never force the individual to engage in an unwanted activity. Remember, keep choice making a positive experience! Use the next choice opportunity to offer the alternative option.

Sigafoos, Roberts, Couzens, and Kerr (1993) taught direct-care staff how to teach choice making resulting in an increase in choice-making responses by people with significant disabilities. Choice options may need to be modified to invite responding.

After presenting this first choice opportunity, you are now ready to repeat several more trials with the same choice pair. Create opportunities for choice making and keep the learner interested by using the small-portion or the turn-taking strategy identified during preparation. Teach choice making by repeating steps 2 to 7 for each choice trial (see Table 2); sampling is not necessary after the first trial. After each choice trial, be sure to vary the position of the options right or left. Continue to present choice trials as long as the learner seems receptive to another opportunity.

Summary

At this point in the process, you should be (a) teaching choice making in two or three routines occurring three to five times per week, (b) presenting multiple choice opportunities for the same choice pair in each routine activity, and (c) teaching choice-making responses following the steps outlined in Table 2.

Evaluate Success

The purpose of this final component is to evaluate how successful you are at teaching beginning choice-making skills.

Two Questions

We evaluate success by asking two questions: (a) Can the learner make independent choice selections? (b) Is the learner making purposeful

Table 3

Component 3: Evaluate Success

1. **Conduct weekly or biweekly probes.**

   a. Choose 10 choice opportunities for each choice pair.

   b. Record the number of independent choice responses.

   c. Record the number of times each option is selected.

2. **Success Outcomes:**

   a. Chooses independently in 80% of the opportunities within at least one choice pair.

   b. Demonstrates preference: Selects one option within at least one pair in 80% or more of the opportunities.

hoice selections? Answering the first question is traightforward. If the learner is choosing without rompts, your teaching is successful. The second uestion is more difficult to answer. Purposeful hoice making can be determined only by bserving preference (i.e., whether the learner hooses one option more frequently than the ther). While some people may "choose" to vary eir responses between options, we cannot be ure that a beginner's responses are purposeful ntil a preference for at least one option has been emonstrated.

Weekly Probes

o answer these evaluation questions, we recomend conducting weekly or biweekly assessment

probes. The steps and outcomes for the assessment are located in Table 3.

Begin the assessment by selecting 10 consecutive choice opportunities (teaching trials) for each targeted choice pair. Choice opportunities may be spread out over several days. Each time the learner makes an independent choice response, record a "+" on a data collection sheet of your choice. Also record the option selected by recording its initial. If the choice response is prompted, record "P." Do not record the name of the selected item for prompted choice responses. Continue to record until 10 consecutive opportunities are completed for each choice pair. An example of a completed data sheet is shown in Figure 2.

Once your assessment is completed, calculate percentages for both independent responses and choice selections. To do so, tally up the number of independent choice responses (or choice selections) within each choice pair and divide by 10.

Because independent choice responses and preference selections are highly influenced by the learner's motivation, we recommend the following minimum outcome measures for success. Success for *independent* choice responses is met when the learner can make independent selections on 80% of the choice opportunities within at least one choice pair. Success for purposeful choice making is determined when the learner selects at least one option within at least one choice pair 80% of the time.

When the learner has successfully met these outcomes, you are ready to expand and extend choice-making opportunities. If the learner has not yet met success, continue teaching until success has been achieved. Be patient. Beginning choice-making skills may take some time to develop.

Troubleshooting

Across weekly probes, you should be encouraged by noticing that the learner is making more and more independent choice responses, showing preferences for particular options. But sometimes you will run into glitches that seem to delay progress. Here are three trouble areas and recommended solutions.

The learner seems interested in choice making on some days, but not on others. It is common for learner interests to vary across days. Sometimes learners are tired or just not in the mood for a particular activity. If you know that the learner still enjoys the choice options but doesn't seem interested on a particular day, skip teaching that day. There will be other opportunities. Remember, keep choice making positive, never force participation.

The learner seems to lose interest in a choice pair(s) after several days of teaching. This problem is more serious than the first; it may suggest that the learner has become bored with the options. If the individual is not motivated to make a choice selection, then you can't teach choice making. The solution is to reconsider learner likes and change the choice options.

To prevent boredom, it may be possible to vary choice options at the onset of instruction. This will require a larger pool of liked items to choose from than originally described. If you can identify several liked items for each routine, it may be possible to vary the choice options across days. However, evaluation must be done within the same choice pairs to determine purposeful choice making.

The learner does not demonstrate a preference for any option. In some cases, learners will learn to make independent choice selections but fail to indicate a preference for any of the options. You may observe the learner always choosing the option to the right or the left (which may suggest a lack of interest for both options) or alternating choice selections between options (which may suggest that the learner is making active choices, but likes both options equally). As discussed, you cannot be sure that the individual making purposeful choice selections until you observe a preference for at least one option.

One solution is to maximize the differences between the options. Either introduce a new, highly motivating favorite or include a disliked option in the choice pair. By presenting contrasting options, you are trying to create a condition that will motivate the learner to choose just one option consistently regardless of its left or right position. You need only to know that the individual can indicate a preference. Thereafter, alternating selections between options should be interpreted as the learner's choice!

Expanding Choice-Making Skills

Some learners have difficulty using or generalizing their new choice-making skills across other choice pairs, settings, or activities that differ from those in which they were trained. As soon as the learner demonstrates reliable choice selections within one choice pair, quickly introduce other choice pairs in different activities and settings. Is the learner making choices in these different situations? If so, you are ready to expand greatly choice opportunities by providing a variety of options across activities throughout the day (see chapter 4). If not, you may need to continue to teach choice making in a few different situations until the learner demonstrates independent, purposeful choice making and generalizes to new situations.

With some adaptations, the basic teaching

steps outlined in Table 2 can also be used to expand choice-making skills. The learner may be taught how to respond to a wider array of options containing three or more items or how to respond to options represented by a different symbolic system (e.g., pictures, spoken words, or objects representing activities, such as a towel for swimming) for maximum flexibility and even greater choice opportunities. Once you understand the process of how choice making is taught, you can be creative in opening up new teaching possibilities.

Illustrated Case

Danielle is a 7-year-old student with severe cognitive and physical limitations. She sits in a wheelchair unable to use her arms or legs with any coordinated fluency. Although she has no formal system of communication, her teacher, Mrs. Johnson, and her mother are attentive to Danielle's subtle cues for indicating likes and dislikes. Danielle spent years in and out of hospitals. As a result, her mother and her teachers fell naturally into care-giving roles, responsive to Danielle's every need, but inadvertently preempting opportunities for Danielle to self-direct. *It is time,* Mrs. Johnson thought, *that we start to teach Danielle how to influence her environment.*

In preparing to present choice opportunities, Mrs. Johnson first needed to identify several foods, objects, or activities that Danielle enjoyed. In consultation with Danielle's mother, Mrs. Johnson identified how she knew that Danielle liked something. When Danielle wanted an object, she appeared to turn her head toward it and look expectantly at it. Once engaged in an activity, she expressed enjoyment by relaxing her body, smiling, and generally cooperating with physical guidance. When she really enjoyed an activity, she would throw her head back, kick her feet, and squeal with delight. By contrast, when Danielle did not like something, she would stiffen her body and turn her head away as if to get as far away from the object or activity as possible.

Using these approach/rejection behaviors to guide them, Mrs. Johnson and Danielle's mother identified several highly desired options that could be presented in a classroom. They included Michael Jackson music, a battery-operated mechanical penguin toy (five penguins march up a ladder, slide down a curvy slide, then march up again), grape juice, and watermelon-scented soap. Next, Mrs. Johnson identified a choice-making response that Danielle could use to signal her selections. Because reaching or pointing would be difficult for Danielle, Mrs. Johnson thought that the most efficient choice response (and one that was generally understood by others) was to teach Danielle to use a response that she was already capable of performing. She defined a choice response as follows: "When presented with two options, Danielle will indicate a choice by turning her head toward an object and looking at it for about 2 seconds."

Still preparing for choice opportunities, Mrs. Johnson needed to form choice pairs, identify classroom activities in which to teach choice making, and consider how to present multiple choice opportunities in each activity while still maintaining Danielle's interest. She considered all three steps simultaneously.

The first choice pair, a Michael Jackson tape (placed in a portable cassette player with headphones) and the marching penguins, would be presented during the classroom free period occurring three or four times per week. Using a turn-taking strategy, Mrs. Johnson planned to make a game out of presenting a choice between these two options, letting Danielle listen or watch for a while, then stopping the activity and offering a choice.

Forming a second choice pair, Mrs. Johnson grouped grape juice with milk. She planned to present this choice pair during in-class snack periods by interspersing a choice (sips of milk or of grape juice) between bites of cookie.

Pairing watermelon soap with another option was a bit of a challenge, but Mrs. Johnson decided to pair a plain bar of soap with a liquid watermelon soap stored in a bright green and pink dispenser. In a wash-up routine after snack, Mrs. Johnson planned to offer a choice between washing with the plain soap or the watermelon soap each time she helped Danielle wash a particular body part (e.g., right hand, left hand, face). Snack and wash-up occurred daily.

Mrs. Johnson was now ready to teach choice making in each of the three routines. At first, when presented with a choice pair, Danielle did not know how to respond. But after consistent choice offers, prompting a choice response, and giving Danielle the opportunity to experience her selections, Danielle soon learned how to make choices and, more important, what choice making was all about.

Using the free activity period as an example, teaching went something like this. Mrs. Johnson started the activity by encouraging Danielle to sample each option. "Look what I have today. You can listen to Michael Jackson!" Mrs. Johnson placed the headphones over Danielle's ears, allowing her to sample a tune. Danielle squealed with delight as Mrs. Johnson did her impression of Michael Jackson. "Or you can play with the penguins." Mrs. Johnson turned on the toy, and watched Danielle stare with interest. Next, Mrs. Johnson placed options on Danielle's lap tray left to right. "Which one do you want to play with? The penguins or Michael?" As she labeled the

options, she pointed to them to direct Danielle's scanning. She waited 5 seconds for Danielle to indicate a choice, but Danielle just looked at Mrs. Johnson. "Use your eyes to tell me what you want." Mrs. Johnson gently turned Danielle's head (physical prompt) toward the cassette tape saying, "There, you told me you want Michael Jackson." She then removed the penguins and placed the headphones on Danielle.

After a minute Mrs. Johnson stopped the tape and presented a second choice opportunity, but this time alternated the placement of the options. Danielle again did not make an independent choice response. Assuming that Danielle wanted to continue with Michael Jackson, she prompted Danielle to make this choice selection. But when she was about to place the headphones on Danielle, Danielle threw her head back and tightened her body. "Oh, you don't want to listen to Michael anymore. What do you want to do?" Mrs. Johnson immediately took this opportunity to offer a choice. "Michael Jackson or the penguins?" This time, Danielle turned toward the penguins and looked at it. "Great! You told me what you wanted by yourself!" Mrs. Johnson turned on the penguins, taking the Michael Jackson tape away. Danielle threw her head back and smiled.

Teaching choice making in each of the three classroom activities continued similarly. On days when Danielle did not appear to be particularly interested in a choice pair, Mrs. Johnson did not present choice opportunities for that pair knowing there would be other opportunities to present Danielle's favorites.

Once a week Mrs. Johnson collected data on Danielle's choice responses and independent choice selections for 10 consecutive choice opportunities within each choice pair. After three weekly probes, Mrs. Johnson noticed an encour-

Figure 2

Sample Data Sheet for
Evaluating Choice Making

Student: Danielle

Behavior: Choice-Making Responses

Week of: 11/13

Key: + = Self-Selected Activity

P = Prompted to Select Activity

	Choice Pair 1			Choice Pair 2		Choice Pair 3	
Trial	Marching Penguins	Michael Jackson	Milk	Grape Juice	Watermelon Soap	Plain Soap
1		P		P	P	
2	P		P			P
3		+	+			+
4	+		+		+	
5		+	+		+	
6	+		+		+	
7	+		+		+	
8	+		+		+	
9	+		+		+	
10	+		+		+	
Percentage of Self-Selected Choices	60%	20%	`80%	0%	70%	10%

ging pattern. Each week Danielle made more ndependent choice responses, and preferences or particular options were emerging. During free •eriod Danielle was making independent choices ♦0% of the time, but she did not demonstrate a trong preference for either the penguins or the ✓lichael Jackson tape, choosing the penguins ▪bout 60% of the time.

Although Danielle's choices appeared •urposeful, Mrs. Johnson could not be sure, so he changed the choice options to maximize their lifferences. Over the next several days, Danielle

was offered a choice between the penguins and a less desired leisure activity—picture cards. By the end of the week, Danielle not only continued to make independent choices, but also demonstrated a strong preference for the penguins, choosing them 90% of the time. Purposeful, independent choice making emerged in the other activities as well. Danielle consistently chose the watermelon-scented soap over the plain soap for washing and surprisingly milk over grape juice during snack.

Because Danielle could make independent

choices across different choice pairs, Mrs. Johnson felt confident that Danielle could use her choice-making skills across different types of options. But she wanted to assess whether Danielle would make choices in different settings. Mrs. Johnson presented the drink options in the lunchroom at school and asked Danielle's mother to present the leisure and soap options at home. Danielle still responded to these choice opportu-nities even in these different settings.

Danielle has now demonstrated basic skills in choice making. She can make independent and purposeful selections. Mrs. Johnson is ready to expand Danielle's choice-making opportunities throughout the day across a wide variety of options.

Embedding Choice Opportunities Across Daily Routines

The primary strategy for embedding choice making involves analyzing daily routines and identifying choice opportunities that can be offered.

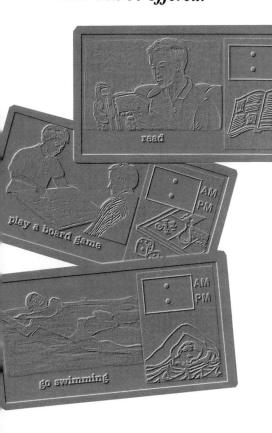

Once learners know how to make basic choices, instructors should ensure that opportunities for choice making are made available throughout the day. In this chapter, we describe a systematic approach for embedding multiple, diverse choice opportunities across and within daily routines.[1] Expanding choice opportunities across the day maximizes learner control and gives learners the opportunity to express preferences across many different situations. It also provides learners with the opportunity to practice, refine, and expand their newly acquired choice-making skills.

The primary strategy for embedding choice making involves analyzing daily routines and identifying different types of choice opportunities that can be offered. The specific steps are outlined in Table 4. The approach is systematic to ensure that meaningful choice options are presented regularly. This is especially critical for people with severe cognitive

> "For choice making to be meaningful to an individual, opportunities must be available throughout the day in all contexts and include a range of choices beyond just a simple choice of two materials within an activity."
>
> —Brown, Belz, Corsi, & Wenig (1993)

disabilities for whom choices may be infrequent or even overlooked. Once you are familiar with the different types of choice options and how to present choices throughout the day, you may use a more informal approach for planning.

Steps for Embedding Choice Opportunities

Identify Daily Routines

Think about the routines or activities that the individual typically engages in each day; list them according to school, home, or community settings. School routines include arrival, opening session (e.g., discuss daily schedules, weather, specials), time at individualized work stations, snack, and small-group reading. Home routines include wake-up/getting dressed, breakfast, arrival from school or work, leisure, dinner preparation, chores, and getting ready for bed.

Identify Choice Options

The second step is to identify the types of choice options that can be made available within each routine. In chapter 3 two types of options (choices between activities and between materials) were described. However, as shown in Table 5, many different types of choices can be considered.

Choice options can be broken down into two broad categories, *between-activities options* and *within-activity options.* Between-activities options offer a choice of activities or tasks within routines. For example, during a work time in a classroom, a student could be offered a choice among math, reading, or spelling assignments. During a spelling period, the student could be offered a choice of writing spelling words or playing hang-man with a partner. At home, between-activities choices for a dinner cleanup routine might include clearing the table, stacking the dishwasher, or taking out the trash.

Once an activity is selected, additional *within*-activity options can be presented by offering a choice of materials; of whether or not to participate; of when to complete the activity; of with whom and where to complete the activity; and of when to terminate the activity. Within-activity choices can be powerful motivators for participation and are especially needed when between-activities options cannot be offered. Examples of within-activity options for a math assignment include a choice of worksheets to complete; a choice of where to sit (e.g., desk or table), or a choice of different-colored pencils.

Table 5

Types and Examples of Choice Options

TYPE OF CHOICE	HOME	SCHOOL	QUESTION FORMAT
Between Activities: Provide a choice between two or more activities during a routine.	**Dinner:** Cook dinner or set the table **Leisure:** Go to the movies or go to the park	**Academics:** Math or reading **Gym:** Basketball or baseball	**Closed:** Would you like to do your math or reading? **Open:** Which subject would you like to do?
Materials: Provide a choice between two or more items within a specific task.	**Dressing:** Pants or dress **Breakfast:** Cereal or oatmeal **Bath:** Shower or bath tub	**Snack:** Cookies or crackers **Math:** Addition flashcards or facts worksheet **Reading:** Options between two stories	**Closed:** Would you like to wear pants or a dress? **Open:** What would you like to wear today?
Refusal: Before beginning a task, provide a choice of whether or not to participate.	**Dinner:** Would you like to set the table or not? **Leisure:** Would you like to go out or not?	**Snack:** Would you like a snack or not?	
Who: At beginning of a task, provide a choice of whom to work or play with.	**Leisure:** Would you like to go to the park with Jen or Rob?	**Snack:** Would you like to eat a snack with Jeff or Rick?	**Closed:** Same **Open:** With whom would you like to have a snack?
Where: At beginning of a task, provide a choice of where to do the activity.	**Household:** Would you like to iron in the laundry room or the living room?	**Academics:** Would you like to complete your work at your desk or the table?	**Closed:** Same **Open:** Where would you like to do your work?
When: Provide a choice of when to participate in an activity.	**Leisure:** Would you like to go out before or after dinner?	**Academics:** Would you like to do your math now or after lunch?	**Closed:** Same **Open:** When would you like to go out?
Terminate: Periodically during the task, provide the choice to quit.	**Leisure:** Let me know when you want to stop.	**Academics:** Let me know when you need a break.	**Closed:** Do you want to stop or continue? **Open:** Let me know when you're done.

Table 6
Individualized Choices Within a Vacuuming Activity

STEPS OF THE ACTIVITY	CHOICE OPTION PRESENTED
1. Takes vacuum to room.	1. Would you like to take the vacuum to the porch or the living room?
2. Plugs vacuum into outlet.	2. Would you like to use the outlet on this wall or that wall?
3. Gets carpet deodorizer.	3. Would you like to use Country Air or Herbal Scent?
4. Sprinkles deodorizer on carpet.	4. Would you like to start sprinkling the deodorizer by the table or the chair?
5. Begins vacuuming area.	5. Would you like to begin vacuuming by the chair or the table?

Options within a home-dusting activity include a choice of rooms, a choice of furniture to dust, and a choice of dusting materials. (See Table 6 for additional choice examples).

When selecting choice options, consider the following factors. First, be certain to offer only those options you can honor immediately. If you cannot honor an option, it is best not to present it. Second, consider the nature of the activity. Is the choice option appropriate or feasible to that activity? Offering a child a choice of whether or not to take seizure medication usually is not appropriate. Other within-activity choices, such as taking the medication with Mommy or Daddy or chasing down the medicine with juice or jelly, are more appropriate choice alternatives and may also add incentives to engage in a disliked but necessary activity. Third, select options based on the individual's known preferences wherever possible. Remember, choice is not meaningful unless it results in a preferred outcome.

Select a Choice Format

Once you have identified choice options, the next step is to *select a choice format* for presenting options. Choices can be presented in either a closed- or open-question format. A closed-question format, such as "Do you want to set the table or take out the trash?" specifies two or more options for the individual. Closed formats are useful when learners are unaware of their options, have difficulty expressing them, or when it is necessary to communicate that "these are your only options." By contrast, an open-question format gives learners the opportunity to generate

heir own options. Examples include "Where
would you like to sit?" and "How do you want to
practice your spelling words?" Open questions
provide greater control than closed formats and
are less repetitive assuming someone knows what
his options are. One obvious disadvantage is that
an individual may choose an option that cannot
be honored. However, this situation creates an
excellent opportunity for teaching the art of
negotiation and compromise.

Present Choice Options

After you have systematically considered the types
of choice options that could be presented, the
next step is to present choice options across the
day. Be sure to take into account the individual's
mode of communication. While some learners
may understand their options presented verbally,
others may need to have their options presented
more concretely such as through objects or
pictures.

When presented with a choice, an individual
may respond in one of three ways. First, the
individual may select one of the choice options, in
which case you should honor the response as
soon as possible.

Second, the individual may choose not to
choose at all. If this is the case, you have several
options: (a) you can present new options if you
believe that the original options were not meaningful; (b) you can accept the individual's
decision not to choose and present the same
options at another time; or (c) you can choose an
option for the learner if participation is essential.
Never reprimand or punish the individual for not
choosing. Choice making invites; it does not
coerce.

An individual can make a third response: to
suggest an alternative option, not previously
presented (e.g., when offered a choice of dusting
or vacuuming, the individual chooses washing

dishes). Once learners experience the power of
choice making, expect them to suggest alternative
options. Choice making can foster self-initiation—an important element needed for full
autonomy. Encourage this. As long as the suggested alternatives are appropriate and feasible,
honor these requests as you would other choice-
making responses. If a spontaneous request
cannot be honored, use this as an opportunity to
negotiate other alternatives.

Modify the Choices

Finally, the last step is to modify the choices based
on your observations of the individual's responses. Initially, you will make "best guesses" as
to the number and type of choice opportunities to
present throughout the day. Then once you start
presenting choices, you will want to individualize
the choice according to the learner's abilities and
interests.

As you modify, ask yourself two general
questions. First, *are the types of choice options
appropriate?* To answer, observe whether or not
the individual is making choices. If he or she is
not responding, then modify the options to
include more meaningful alternatives. Failure to
respond may also mean that the individual does
not know how to make choices (in which case
you will need to teach, see chapter 3) or does not
understand the choice format (in which case you
could change the mode of presentation). If the
learner is responding, consider introducing novel
choice options as a means of expanding experiences and creating new opportunities for choice
making.

Second, ask yourself if *the number of choice
opportunities is appropriate.* An individual
frequently suggesting alternative options to the
ones you are presenting may be seeking more
opportunities for choice making or would prefer
an open-choice format. If the individual is

consistently choosing the same choice option and appears a bit annoyed with your questions (e.g., "Do you want orange juice or grape juice?" for the umpteenth time), stop presenting a choice here. Instead, build preferences into daily routines by simply making them available (e.g., keep grape juice stocked in the refrigerator).

Opportunities for choice should be made available throughout the day, but note that "more choices" do not necessarily mean "better choices." Some people like to make a few but highly meaningful choices each day, such as deciding what activities to engage in. For others, this is not enough; they would prefer making multiple choices during the course of each activity. Follow the individual's lead and decide.

Summary

At this point, you should have identified various types of choice options that can be presented across and within daily routines and activities. Following the outline in Table 4 as a guide, present choice opportunities across the day, in a format appropriately matched to the nature of the activity and the individual's communication style. Modify choice opportunities based on the individual's responses.

When students with emotional and behavioral challenges were provided with a variety of task options within academic subjects, their participation increased substantially.

—Dunlap & Colleagues (1994)

Case Illustration in a Classroom

Rick is a 10-year-old student with moderate cognitive disabilities. He communicates using three- to five-word sentences and has just recently been taught how to make simple choices by his teacher Ms. New. Now that Rick can clearly make his preferences known through choice, Ms. New believes it is important to give Rick a way to have greater control over the activities occurring during his school day. What's more, by embedding choices throughout his classroom routines, Rick will have the opportunity to practice, refine, and expand his choice-making skills.

To get started, Ms. New identified Rick's daily routines and the associated activities within each. Broadly defined, Rick's daily routines included arrival, morning academics, lunch, leisure, afternoon academics, and departure.

Once she identified these basic routines, Ms. New selected the types of choice options that would be feasible to offer to Rick. In selecting the options, Ms. New believed it was important to provide choices of refusal only during certain activities. Rick was working quite hard at his academics this year. An option to refuse math or reading assignments can be detrimental to his education. Instead, during academic routines, Ms. New offered Rick a choice of when to complete specific assignments during the morning and afternoon work periods. This choice option gave Rick control over sequencing assignments without jeopardizing learning. Whenever possible, Ms. New offered Rick additional within-activity choices by giving him options of different types of work assignments or materials (e.g., drill on the computer or with flash cards), places to work, and peers to work with. There were many ways to achieve the same

Figure 3
Choice Options for Rick

RICK'S ROUTINE	CHOICE OPTIONS
Arrival	**Who:** Walk in with aide or teacher **Where:** Enter building through one of two doors
Morning Academics	**Between Activities:** Reading or math **Materials:** Spelling bingo or flashcards **Who:** Work alone or with a classmate **Where:** Complete activity at desk or table
Lunch	**Materials:** Prepare food or drink first **Termination:** Free to quit when ready **Who:** Eat alone, with classmate or teacher **Where:** Option between different seats
Leisure	**Between:** Board game or puzzle **Materials:** Monopoly or Mouse Trap **Refusal:** Free to participate or not **Termination:** Free to stop when ready **Who:** Play game with Jen or Rob **Where:** Play game at table or desk
Afternoon Academics	**Materials:** Math board game or flashcards **Who:** Work alone or with classmate **Where:** Complete activity at desk or table
Departure	**Who:** Walk out with aide or teacher **Where:** Leave the building through one of two doors

academic objectives and keep learning fun! Options to refuse participation were provided during leisure and lunch routines, giving Rick further control over the events in his school day. Additional examples of the types of choice options presented to Rick are shown in Figure 3.

Once Ms. New identified possible choice options for each routine, she decided to present the choices in a closed-question format in all activities except leisure. Rick seemed well aware of his leisure options but would be unable to generate appropriate options for academic subjects.

As planned, Ms. New presented Rick with his choice options throughout the day in either a closed- or open-question format for several days. During this time, she carefully observed Rick's choice responses so that she could make any necessary modifications. After a week Ms. New decided that some changes were needed.

Rick was having difficulty understanding his options for academic subjects when they were presented verbally to him. To modify the choice format, Ms. New showed him an example of each option, such as a specific activity sheet or an assignment in a workbook, until he learned the names of the different types of tasks. During lunch Ms. New noticed that Rick would offer alternatives to the offered options. For example, if given a choice of where to sit during lunch, he would point to yet another seat. Ms. New modified her choice format during lunch by providing open questions. In the final modification, Ms. New introduced beginning negotiation skills. During leisure time Rick would frequently choose activities that other students were playing with. Ms. New used these opportunities to offer Rick other options while he waited for materials to become available.

Individualizing Choice Based on Problem Behaviors

Problem behaviors can sometimes provide clues for individualizing choice opportunities in meaningful ways. Some people may engage in problem behaviors to avoid participating in certain activities. In this case consider presenting many options among activities and tasks. Through choice making, the individual can reject an activity appropriately without having to engage in problem behaviors; at the same time she can indicate a suitable alternative. Providing within-activity choices also may be helpful for reducing the unpleasantness of a task. Options such as where to sit, what materials to use, and when to engage in an activity can result in making a disliked activity enjoyable.

Other people who are motivated by control may engage in problem behaviors because they do not like being told what to do. In such cases consider providing many between- and within-activities choices. By providing many multiple choices, the individual should get the sense that he or she is leading or at least "copiloting" the activity.

The following case illustrates how choice making was individualized based on one man's problem behaviors.

Case Illustration: Individualizing Choice Based on Problem Behaviors

Al, a 50-year-old with severe cognitive disabilities, lived in a group home in the community. He spoke in one- to three-word sentences, but only people who knew him well could understand him. Al enjoyed many community activities. He had the skills to participate in a wide variety of household and self-care routines. But to participate, Al frequently required prompts to initiate activities and to move to the next step in his routines. This had created a problem. Al did not like to be told what to do.

At first Al's support staff did not recognize his need for control. Whenever they prompted him to engage in a household activity, Al responded by yelling, cursing, breaking objects, and sometimes showing aggression toward others. His protests were perplexing, because he protested even during activities he enjoyed very much. For example, quite often he would grab a staff member's hand, lead her to the kitchen, and say, "Let's bake." However, during the course of the baking, when Al was directed to break the eggs into the bowl, Al angrily stormed out of the kitchen. It was the same during community activities. The staff, believing they were honoring Al's choices not to participate, soon stopped prompting Al to engage in activities. As a result, he sat in his room for increasingly longer periods just listening to his radio.

"This is absurd," cried Jeff, the staff person closest to Al. "Al is unhappy. Certainly choice making does not mean that we give up and let Al waste away alone in his room." The staff called a team meeting. After lengthy discussions about when Al would protest, they concluded that Al would engage in problem behaviors in most any

30

ctivity; preferred or not preferred it didn't matter. It wasn't the activity he was refusing but the way he was being prompted.

The staff's first solution was to offer Al between-activities options within his daily routines. That was the easy part. Between-activities options would give Al control over what to do and the opportunity to refuse activities without having to protest. But what about when Al needed prompts during the course of an activity? He could rarely complete an activity without being given some direction. Beginning with several household activities Al appeared to enjoy, the staff wrote down the specific steps for which Al might need prompts. Then for each step, they brainstormed how they could translate prompts into a choice opportunity. An example for a vacuuming activity is shown in Table 6. Each choice opportunity (e.g., "Would you like to take the vacuum cleaner to the living room or the porch?") served as a prompt to begin a step, while at the same time gave Al control over the direction of the activity.

Some choice options needed modification. In the baking activity, Al consistently refused to wash his hands before starting, even though he was given a choice of washing with two kinds of soaps. Although the staff could honor Al's choice not to wash, they saw this step as being essential, because Al did not have good hygiene habits. *I wonder why Al refuses to wash his hands,* thought Jeff. *Al's hands are often dry and chapped. Perhaps the soap and water irritates them.* Al was offered new options. He could choose to wash at the sink or use a moist towelette to clean his hands. Al almost always chose the towelettes. "What a simple solution," said Jeff, "if only Al could have told us what was bothering him, we could have solved this long ago."

As Al was offered more and more choices, he eagerly participated in more household and community activities. He also learned to say no appropriately without engaging in problem behaviors. Moreover, to the surprise of staff, he began to initiate many more activities. When he finished baking, he initiated cleanup. When he vacuumed one room, he initiated another. Contrary to the staff's original beliefs, Al truly enjoyed participating in his home *when he* was in control.

[1] In addition to the two research foundations for this chapter, Bambara, Koger, Katzer, & Davenport (1995) and Dunlap et al. (1994), many of the concepts related to analyzing daily routines and embedding diverse choice opportunities are based on an article by Brown, Belz, Corsi, & Wenig (1993). (See bibliography for full citation.) Table 5 was adapted from Dr. Brown's work in defining and analyzing choice opportunities.

*S*elf-Scheduling as a Choice-Making Strategy

Shared planning, ongoing discussion, and negotiation are the basic tools used to guide self-scheduling.

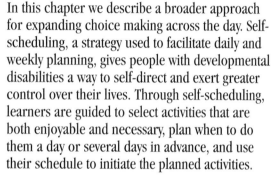

In this chapter we describe a broader approach for expanding choice making across the day. Self-scheduling, a strategy used to facilitate daily and weekly planning, gives people with developmental disabilities a way to self-direct and exert greater control over their lives. Through self-scheduling, learners are guided to select activities that are both enjoyable and necessary, plan when to do them a day or several days in advance, and use their schedule to initiate the planned activities.

Shared planning, ongoing discussion, and negotiation are the basic tools used to guide self-scheduling. A wide array of activity options are presented through pictures. Through discussion and negotiation, the individual identifies what to do and places it on a picture calendar. Once the calendar is complete, the person is guided to refer to the schedule to initiate activities, similar to the way readers refer to things-to-do lists or week-at-a-glance organizers.

Self-scheduling expands choice and control in several ways. First, by self-scheduling, learners can select both the sequence and the nature of daily events over extended periods. Self-scheduling allows someone to choose what to do later in the day or in the week. This is especially critical for activities that require advanced planning such as having friends over for dinner. Second, using pictured activities expands the number of choice options that can be presented at one time. By flipping through the pictures, learners are reminded about the wide array of activities that can be made available. Third, self-scheduling fosters self-initiation. Once placed on a calendar, pictured activities serve as cues for "what to do," lessening dependence on others for direction. For people motivated by control, this aspect is a real plus. Finally, self-scheduling moves beyond simple choice making and encourages self-determination by giving people a strategy for identifying what to do and how or when to do it.

Learner Prerequisites and Self-Scheduling Overview

There are many strategies for helping people to plan their day. The approach we describe requires skills in basic choice making and picture reading (e.g., being able to interpret the depicted object and action). In addition, learners should be able to identify the days of week and understand basic time concepts such as today, tomorrow, before, and after.

Self-scheduling involves three components: (1) prepare for scheduling, (b) create a schedule, and (c) follow the schedule (see Table 7). Your goal will be to assist the learner to (a) schedule three to five activities a day from 2 to 7 days in advance, (b) initiate the activities depicted in the calendar, and (c) revise the schedule as needed. We chose to emphasize home

> When three adults with developmental disabilities were taught how to self-schedule their leisure activities, their self-direction increased. Further, the adults engaged in many more new activities than previously.
>
> —Bambara & Ager (1992)

Table 7

Strategy for Training Self-Scheduling

Prepare for Scheduling

1. Identify time periods to schedule.
2. Identify activity options.
   a. "Things I like to do."
   b. "Things I need to do."
3. Prepare picture cards.
4. Design an activity calendar.

Create a Schedule

1. Present choice options.
2. Guide choice making.
3. Place activity cards on the calendar.
4. Expand self-scheduling across days.

Follow the Schedule

5. Prompt looking at the calendar.
6. Encourage self-initiations.
7. Review and modify.

---

settings because of their inherent flexibility. Once the steps within each component are described, we will suggest ways to expand self-scheduling and how it might be adapted for school settings.

Prepare for Scheduling

In this first component, begin by preparing the materials needed for self-scheduling: illustrated activity cards and an activity calendar. Start by *identifying time periods* during the day for scheduling. Scheduling all possible activities all day long, every day, is neither practical nor easible. Rather, select several time slots for cheduling that will allow the most flexibility for hoice making. The most common time slots for cheduling home activities are late afternoons after school/work until dinner), early evenings after dinner until bedtime), and early afternoons lunch until dinner) on weekends.

Next, *identify activity options* that can be made available for choice making. It is helpful to ivide activities into two categories. "Things I like o do" refers to in-home and community leisure ptions such as painting, calling friends, going to he movies, or eating out. "Things I have to do" efers to daily living activities, such as personal are (e.g., bathing, going to the dentist), house-old chores (e.g., cleaning the kitchen), and ersonal management (e.g., budgeting, paying ills). Be sure to identify a wide array of possible ctivities including routine activities that occur requently during the week (e.g., watching T.V.), s well as special activities that occur occasionally e.g., eating out, visiting friends). But remember, ptions must be motivating enough to invite a hoice response and should be based on learner references.

Once the activities are identified, *prepare icture cards* to represent each one. You can reate your own hand-drawn illustrations, cut ctures from a magazine, take photographs, or se commercially produced picture cards. hatever you use, be sure that the learner can ead" the picture format (e.g., line drawings rsus photos) and knows what each activity card eans. For example, some learners cannot terpret line drawings, but can readily read otographs of actual objects. Before you start heduling, be sure that the learner can identify label each activity card. As an alternative to ctures, you may use word cards for readers.

Now you are ready to *design an activity calendar.* Activity calendars should clearly illustrate up to a week of scheduled activities in a picture book or wall-chart format. Picture-book activity calendars can be made using a photo album with clear plastic slots to hold the activity cards, about six to eight slots per page. The two facing pages in an open book can represent one day; turn the page for the next day, and so on. A wall chart, constructed out of poster board, can illustrate activities across the entire week, like a week-at-a-glance organizer. Here activity cards are sequenced in vertical columns, one for each day of the week, and affixed with Velcro for easy reshuffling. A picture-book activity calendar is illustrated in Figure 4.

Calendars should be clearly labeled with each day of the week. You can use arrows or another marker to signify "today." Because many people with developmental disabilities cannot read or tell time, use illustrated time markers to designate daily routines that occur approximately the same time each day. Examples of time markers include illustrations of arriving home from work or school, eating dinner, and going to bed. By spacing the markers within a day on a calendar, learners can schedule activities "before" or "after" these set routines (e.g., "Do you want to go to the store before or after dinner?"), and, once scheduled, get a sense of when planned activities will be occurring during the day.

Summary

By the end of this component you should have at hand all the materials needed for self-scheduling, including activity cards for choice making and an activity calendar for scheduling. Modify as you go along, adding new cards for new activity options. You are now ready to help the learner to self-schedule.

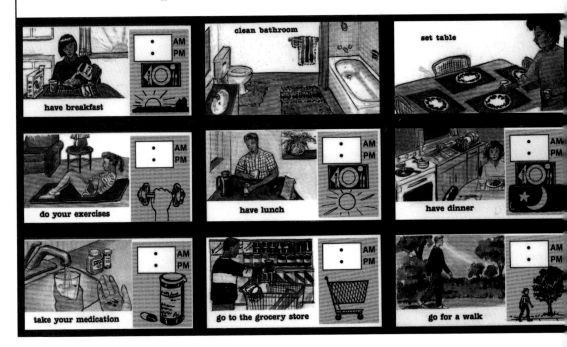

Figure 4

Sample Picture-Book Activity Calendar

have breakfast · AM · PM

clean bathroom

set table

do your exercises · AM · PM

have lunch · AM · PM

have dinner · AM · PM

take your medication · AM · PM

go to the grocery store · AM · PM

go for a walk · AM · PM

Create a Schedule

Self-scheduling is conducted in the context of discussion and shared decision making in which you present choice options, guide the learner to decide what to do and when to do it, and place the activity cards on the calendar. Begin, by scheduling one day at a time, approximately three to five activities for each time period. Once the individual draws an association between the scheduled activities and the day's events, slowly expand scheduling across several days up to a week at a time.

To get started, choose a comfortable time to schedule with the learner. *Present choice options* for the first day by laying out several activity cards in each choice category: (a) "Things I want to do" and (b) "Things I need to do." The number of options to present will depend on several factors including (a) the learner's ability to attend to multiple options, (b) the learner's preference for choice making (e.g., some people are comfortable with many options, while others prefer no more than two or three at a time), and (c) your ability to honor the choice request.

Next, *guide choice making* by asking three important choice questions: (a) "What would you like to do?" (b) "What do you need to do?" and (c) "When would you like to do it?" As you ask these questions, you may offer suggestions. To

cilitate informed decision making, you also may
ffer pros or cons for each choice selection. For
xample, "If you go to the mall after dinner, then
ou will miss your favorite T.V. show. Would you
ke to go this afternoon or skip it today?" Or,
You really ought to go to the bank this afternoon
efore it closes; otherwise you will be out of
oney." Through your suggestions you are
elineating further options and guiding the
dividual to recognize natural constraints. But
emember, the choice is ultimately the learner's.
the individual chooses not to choose, then
espond as you would for any other choice
pportunity (see chapter 4). You may, for
stance, honor the individual's choice not to
oose, offer alternative activity options, or, in
ome cases, choose an activity for the individual
hen appropriate.

As the learner selects activities, guide him to
lace the cards on the calendar in sequence
efore or after the time markers on a given day.
chedule as many activities as appropriate.
nally, expand scheduling across days as soon
the learner understands how to schedule for
e day. Use the same approach as we described
plan for several days or a week at a time. Now
hen you ask, "When would you like to do it?"
ou are asking which day. By scheduling across
ays, you can offer a wider array of choice
ptions and schedule "big" activities that require
dvanced planning or preparation.

ummary

this point you should be helping the learner
hedule activities once a day, and then once for
veral days at a time. Scheduling takes place in
e context of discussion in which you present
ptions, guide choice making, and help the
arner place activity cards on the calendar.

Follow the Schedule

In this last component, you will be guiding the
learner to refer to her calendar, initiate the
planned activities, then revise the schedule as
necessary. First, prompt the learner to *look at the
calendar* during the same routine activity each
day. For example, the learner might be prompted
to look at her calendar while eating her snack
immediately after school. The calendar may be
kept in the kitchen as a visual cue. After a few
days of reminders, wait for independent looking,
then prompt only as needed.

Second, once the learner is looking at the
calendar, discuss the schedule, then wait for the
learner to *self-initiate* by either beginning the
activities independently or indicating what needs
to be done (e.g., "Let's go to the mall"). Initially,
the learner may need several reminders during
the day to start each activity, but he or she should
begin to initiate over time. Remember, even while
prompting initiations, you are still offering choice
making. Learners still have the option to change
their minds.

Finally, in the last step, *review and modify*
the schedule with the learner at the end of each
day. Here you are encouraging the learner to self-
evaluate choices by asking, "Did you do what you
had planned?" If the answer is yes, you may
discuss what was liked about the activities or the
way they were sequenced. Perhaps the same
activities could be scheduled similarly in the
future. If an activity was not done, you may
explore "why not?" Perhaps an activity is disliked.
Discussion may center around how to make it
more enjoyable. Perhaps time was inappropriate
(e.g., too tired to clean during the evening).
Discussion may center on how the activity may be
scheduled differently in the future. After discussion, offer the opportunity to revise the calendar
by adding, removing, or rescheduling activities
across the next several days.

Summary

At this point, you should have implemented all three components of self-scheduling. Creating and following a schedule become permanent ongoing strategies for expanding learner choice and control. In this last component, you should be guiding the learner to refer to the calendar and to initiate activities. Finally, by reviewing completed activities each day, you help the learner self-evaluate and modify his schedule as needed.

The following case illustrates how self-scheduling was used by one young man in his home.

Illustrated Case

Ben, a 22-year-old recent high school graduate, had just moved into the apartment he shared with two other men. Ben contracted for staff support for about 5 hours each day for help with transportation, general problem solving, and the daily management of his household and community activities.

Ben was quite adept at performing tasks of daily living and traveled independently in his community. He also had a strong sense of independence. This was his home and nobody was going to tell him what to do.

The first several months of Ben's relationship with his support staff was tense, to say the least. Ben was highly motivated to initiate and engage in community leisure activities, but he was so involved in his leisure pursuits that he did not allot time for essential activities such as washing his clothes, showering, banking, or shopping. This caused severe problems for Ben. His employer complained about his poor grooming habits, threatening to fire him. Ben would frequently run out of spending money and food, then demand to go to the bank or the store when it was not possible, leaving him angry and frustrated. Seeing his dilemma, support staff attempted to prompt Ben to attend to his daily living needs, but Ben perceived their prompts as nags interfering with what he wanted to do. When staff could not accommodate his immediate requests, such as to go to the bank when it was closed or to go to the amusement park when there was no public transportation on Sunday, Ben viewed the staff as unnecessarily blocking him from doing the things he liked. On the other hand, staff perceived Ben as being unreasonably demanding. Occasionally anger erupted into physical aggression. Few people wanted to work for Ben, and Ben felt he had no need for support staff.

Although Ben had a strong desire to direct his own life, his lack of planning actually worked against him. Robert, a support staff person who decided to stick with Ben, introduced Ben to self-scheduling as a means for Ben to manage his own daily affairs.

Preparation for self-scheduling began with Robert explaining to Ben that he could do more things if he took the time to plan. Together they identified periods for each day that were most appropriate for scheduling (e.g., after work until bedtime on weekdays and after lunch until bedtime on weekends) and identified important activities to be scheduled. Things Ben liked to do included going to the local coffee shop, browsing in the record store, visiting friends, taking guitar lessons, watching his favorite T.V. shows, and going to the amusement park. Things that Ben needed to do included showering, washing clothes, banking, food shopping, housecleaning, paying his bills, and calling his mother once a week.

Robert constructed a wall chart activity calendar out of posterboard, adding Velcro backing to affix activity cards. This week-at-aance format was an excellent choice for Ben, ecause it helped him predict upcoming events nd see that his favorite activities would be rthcoming. Activity cards were made from agazine pictures and actual photographs of ojects in Ben's home or in the community. ultiple copies of the same activity cards were ade for activities that could occur several times r week, such as showering or going to the local ffee shop. As the cards were constructed, obert asked Ben to identify each, making sure at he labeled the activity (e.g., amusement rk) and not just the object in the picture (e.g., ller coaster).

Each night about 20 minutes before Ben's vorite T.V. show, Robert or another assistant lped Ben schedule the next day's activities. They et in the kitchen where the activity chart was sted. Robert began the self-scheduling process laying out all the activity cars on the kitchen ple and asking guiding questions: "What would u like to do tomorrow? What do you need to ? When would you like to do it?" To aid Ben's cision making, Robert offered suggestions for ecific activities or discussed the pros or cons · each activity as Ben selected it. Whenever ssible, Robert guided Ben to recognize natural heduling constraints. For example, Robert couraged Ben to call his friends before plan- ig a visit with them. Before arranging a trip to e amusement park, Robert and Ben looked ough the bus schedule to identify feasible vel times. When a desired activity could not be heduled for the next day, Robert encouraged n to choose an alternative day and to immedi- ly place the activity card on the calendar. This ped to assure Ben that his favorite activities re not being denied.

For activities Ben needed to do but did not essarily prefer to do, Robert suggested times t would not interfere with Ben's leisure activities. Whenever possible, Robert helped Ben see the importance of these necessary activities by linking them to the things that Ben liked to do. "It might be a good idea to do your laundry before you go to the amusement park, so you'll have clean shorts to wear." Once Ben had selected the activities for the next day, he placed the activity cards on the calendar in the order he preferred to do them before or after the time markers for that day.

Learning to follow his schedule came easily for Ben. "When you come home from work and pour your glass of iced tea, or when you eat your lunch on Saturdays and Sundays, take a look at what you have planned." Ben needed to be reminded only a few times before he started to refer to his calendar independently. After Ben reviewed his schedule, Robert waited for Ben to initiate. Ben needed no further reminders to initiate leisure activities but typically required a prompt before he started the necessary activities. If Ben did not initiate a necessary activity as planned, Robert reminded him to look at his calendar. If he still did not initiate, Robert honored Ben's choice not to participate at that time.

Robert encouraged Ben to look at his schedule at the same time each day.

Each evening, just before Ben scheduled the next day's activities, Ben and Robert reviewed the schedule for the current day, this time discussing which activities Ben had or had not participated in. Robert guided Ben to self-evaluate. "What did you enjoy doing today? Would you like to do it again?" If Ben did not initiate an activity, Robert helped him to problem solve. "Why didn't you want to go food shopping? What could you do differently in the future?" Ben was finding it hard to fit showering in his busy schedule. Although he knew why it was important, he did not like getting up early to shower the first thing in the morning. He was usually too tired to shower after watching television at night. Finally, after several days of failed attempts, Ben discovered that the best time to shower was right after dinner, just before watching T.V. and planning his days.

Over the next two months, Ben gradually scheduled activities for the entire week. Decisions about what to do and when to do it became easier as many of the activities fell into routines and as Ben became aware of scheduling constraints. Showering was usually scheduled after dinner each night, guitar lessons on Wednesday afternoons, laundry on Friday evenings, and the amusement park on Saturday afternoons. Activity cards for these set activities remained on the calendar each week.

Ben now uses his calendar to schedule occasional or special activities such as participating in his neighborhood block watch meetings or attending the state fair. New activity cards are added as Ben's interests and daily living needs expand. Although Ben's day-to-day activities have fallen into a routine, nightly scheduled reviews continue. Ben is always presented with the option of rearranging his schedule as new events arise or as he simply changes his mind.

Adaptations

Like all choice-making strategies, self-scheduling is meant to be adapted to the individual learner. Use it flexibly to adapt to a person's skills, abilities, and interests. For example, some people prefer to schedule a week at a time. Others feel more comfortable scheduling a day at a time. Some prefer unchanging schedules; others like

the option of rearranging their routines each week. Some learners may be interested in a two-calendar strategy in which monthly events are pictured on a traditional calendar and daily events are sequenced in a small pocket-sized organizer that can be carried around.

Self-scheduling may be used to foster independent problem solving. Guide learners to discover scheduling constraints rather than telling them directly. For instance, a learner may be guided to arrange her own transportation or call the movie theater to find out when a movie is playing. As the individual is deciding what to do, have her discuss the possible outcomes of choosing whether or not to participate in certain activities.

Self-scheduling may also be adapted for school use. The following brief example illustrates how one teacher used a form of self-scheduling in her classroom.

Brief Classroom Example

Mrs. Jones, teacher of a first-grade inclusion classroom, explained how self-scheduling work in her class. "This is my third year teaching first graders with diverse needs. I needed some way accommodating to a wide range of abilities, so Mr. Nyce, another first-grade teacher, and I developed a learning-center approach. Between our two classrooms we have nine learning centers, one for reading, math, writing, science listening, computers, art, block building, and special themes. The children from both class-rooms go to the centers for about an hour durin the morning and afternoon work sessions. Each center is filled with a variety of activities, indivi alized according to specific skills.

"Each Monday the children are given their own special work assignments for the week. I explained that this is how adults did their work

eir jobs. Assignment sheets are divided into
ust-do' activities and 'free choice.' Under the
ust-do and free-choice categories, I draw a
mbol for each learning center and the number
times a student must attend a center each
eek. At the centers, activities are further indi-
dualized by placing students' names on specific
signments. Children can visit the free-choice
nters as much as they want.

"Once the children are given their assign-
ents, they are free to choose which center they
ant to go to and which assignments to complete
st. I try to give them a choice of assignments in
ch activity center as well. Management is a bit
a problem, so I have rules about the number of
ildren at each center. I also enlist the help of
rent volunteers, teaching assistants, and the
rning support teacher.

"As the children complete their assignments,
ey color in the appropriate symbol on their
signment sheets and place their work in a
folder. I grade both their completed assignments
and their assignment sheets, noting how well they
have met their responsibilities. At the end of the
week, I meet with the students individually. We
discuss their grades, how to improve their
performance, and how to make better use of their
time. Some children were not organizing them-
selves well, hanging out too much in the block
area and not getting their 'must dos' done. For a
while I met with these students each day to help
them plan their morning and afternoon activities."

We asked, "Now that you have been using this
center approach for several months, what do you
think about it?"

"I love it," said Mrs. Jones. "The kids love it,
too. I did it as a way to individualize instruction,
but do you know what I've noticed? There is such
a positive atmosphere in this class, better than any
class I've taught. All of my kids seem happy and
motivated to learn. They really enjoy having the
responsibility to make decisions about their day."

ummary, Questions, and Answers

Use, refine, and adapt these procedures as you discover new choice-making possibilities for people with developmental disabilities.

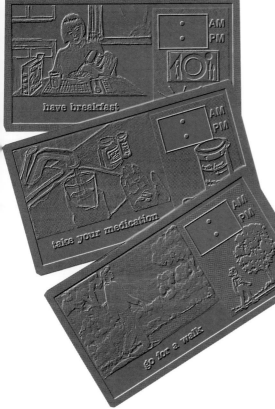

In this book we emphasize the importance of choice making. We offer three research-based strategies for expanding choice making throughout the day. These strategies range from teaching initial choice-making skills to facilitating complex choice making by self-scheduling. By way of summarizing some important points, we address some common questions and concerns.

But I Know What She Prefers

Should I still provide choices when I know what the individual prefers?

Yes. When presented with options, some people will demonstrate a consistent preference for certain tasks, materials, or activities. When this happens, you can build preferences into their daily routines. (We are all comforted knowing that our preferences are made available without having to be asked what we want.) But continue to provide opportunities for choice making by pairing old favorites with new options or by creating completely new choice opportunities.

People's preferences change over time. Choice prevents us from being locked in and becoming bored with old favorites.

Further, choice creates opportunities for control. Remember, some folks resent being told what to do even when they are directed to perform a preferred activity. Customize choice opportunities, by observing and following a learner's responses.

Neglected Activities

When I present choices, the individual avoids engaging in important activities. What should I do?

When offered a choice between activities, one will not be selected. It is integral to the definition of choice making. A common concern is that learners will consistently avoid activities that are essential for learning or participation in community life. To address this, consider two questions. First, is the activity essential? Be sure to evaluate from the individual's perspective and not your own agenda. Does the individual *have to* engage in this particular activity? Are there acceptable alternatives? When evaluated from this perspective, that list of "have tos" is often considerably smaller than first perceived. There may be a countless number of reasonable alternatives. If the activity doesn't have to be done or can be done by someone else in exchange for another activity, such as sharing household chores, then "escape" should not be a concern.

If the activity has to be done (e.g., going to the dentist, taking a shower/bath), the next question is, what specifically is the individual trying to avoid? Often an individual is seeking to avoid only particular aspects of the activity. How can the activity be modified to make it more pleasurable? Consider providing choices *within* the activity. As shown in Al's case (chapter 4), choices within an activity can be used to alter the problem aspect of the activity (e.g., running water irritates chapped hands), while still maintaining its critical outcome (e.g., clean hands).

Delayed Delivery?

What should I do if I cannot honor the individual's choice right away?

Present only those options that you can

honor immediately. Delay delivery, such as during self-scheduling, only when the individual can anticipate that his or her choice will be received eventually. If the individual does not understand waiting, it is best not to present options until a choice can be honored. This is especially critical when teaching initial choice-making skills. If the individual makes a spontaneous choice request that cannot be honored immediately, be honest. you cannot fulfill a request, say no or indicate when you can.

Problem Behaviors Persist

I am presenting many choices throughout the day, but the individual is still engaging in problem behaviors. What should I do?

First and foremost, it is important to recognize that choice making is a basic human right. should not be viewed as just an intervention to reduce problem behaviors. However, as we have stressed, choice making can have a profound effect on reducing challenging behaviors *when problem behaviors are related to the absence choice or control* (e.g., when the individual is forced to engage in a nonpreferred activity or when the individual is told what to do). But then may be other explanations for problem behavio If problem behaviors persist in the presence of rich choice opportunities, explore other reason for their occurrence and pursue other interventions.

Allow Bad Choices?

Should I let the individual make bad choices?

Sometimes a learner will choose an option you know will result in a nonpreferred or poor outcome (e.g., blowing an allowance on one item, leaving no spending money for the rest of the week). As long as the bad choice doesn't

create serious health or safety risks, allow the individual the dignity of learning from his mistakes. You can always temper the experience by explaining possible consequences beforehand or helping the individual to terminate the unpleasant situation. Both good and bad choice selections are important for making informed decisions in the future.

Limited Benefits?

We tried presenting choices, but the individual just doesn't seem interested. Is it possible that certain people just do not benefit from choice making?

No! All people benefit from choice making. It is our responsibility to make choice making work. After being denied opportunities for choice making, it may take time before some people with disabilities recognize the power of their choice selections. Be persistent. If the individual does not seem to catch on initially, troubleshoot by asking the summary questions listed in Table 8. The solutions are addressed throughout this book.

The strategies and the instructional principles described in this book were designed to give you the tools to apply choice making in your own situations. We encourage you to use, refine, and adapt these procedures as you discover new choice-making possibilities for people with developmental disabilities.

Table 8

Summary Trouble-Shooting Questions

1. Does the person know how to make choice selections?

2. Does the person know what options are available? Are options presented in a way that the learner can understand?

3. Has the person had sufficient experience with the options? Does the learner know what the options are?

4. Are options sufficiently motivating to invite a choice response?

5. Do options result in meaningful outcomes? Access to a preferred event or control?

6. Are choices varied? Could the person be bored with the options?

7. Are choices presented in a rich environment that introduces the individual to new experiences and new options?

8. Are choice responses honored immediately? If delayed, does the individual understand waiting?

Bibliography

Bambara, L. M., & Ager, C. (1992). Using self-scheduling to promote self-directed leisure activity in home and community settings. *Journal of The Association for Persons with Severe Handicaps, 17,* 67-76.

Bambara, L. M., Ager, C., & Koger, F. (1994). The effects of choice and task preference on the work performance of adults with severe disabilities. *Journal of Applied Behavior Analysis, 27,* 555-556.

Bambara, L. M., Koger, F., Katzer, T., & Davenport, T. (1995). Embedding choice in daily routines: An experimental case study. *Journal of The Association for Persons with Severe Handicaps, 20,* 185-195.

Brown, F. (1991). Creative daily scheduling: A nonintrusive approach to challenging behaviors in community residences. *Journal of The Association for Persons with Severe Handicaps, 16,* 75-84.

Brown, F., Belz, P., Corsi, L., & Wenig, B. (1993). Choice diversity for people with severe disabilities. *Education and Training in Mental Retardation, 28,* 318-326.

Carr, E. G., Levin, L., McConnachie, G., Carlson, J. I., Kemp, D. C., & Smith, C. E. (1994). *Communication-based intervention for problem behavior: A user's guide for producing positive change.* Baltimore: Paul H. Brookes.

Dunlap, G., dePerczel, C. S., Clarke, S., Wilson, D., Wright, S., White R., & Gomez, A. (1994). Choice making to promote adaptive behavior for students with emotional and behavioral challenges. *Journal of Applied Behavior Analysis, 27,* 505-518.

Dyer, K., Dunlap, G., & Winterling, V. (1990). Effects of choice-making on the serious problem behaviors of students with severe handicaps. *Journal of Applied Behavior Analysis, 23,* 515-524.

Guess, D., Benson, H. A., & Siegel-Causey, E. (1985). Concepts and issues related to choice-making and autonomy among persons with severe disabilities. *Journal of The Association for Persons with Severe Handicaps, 10,* 79-86.

Houghton, J., Bronicki, G. J. B., & Guess, D. (1987). Opportunities to express preferences and make choices among students with severe disabilities in classroom settings. *Journal of The Association for Persons with Severe Handicaps, 12,* 18-27.

Kishi, G., Teelucksingh, B., Zollers, S. P., & Meyer, L. (1988). Daily decision making in community residences: A social comparison of adults with and without mental retardation. *American Journal on Mental Retardation, 92,* 430-435.

Parsons, M. B., McCarn, J. E., & Reid, D. H. (1993). Evaluating and increasing meal-related choices throughout a service setting for people with severe disabilities. *Journal of The Association for Persons with Severe Handicaps, 18,* 253-260.

Parsons, M. B., & Reid, D. H. (1990). Assessing food preferences among persons with profound mental retardation: Providing opportunities to make choices. *Journal of Applied Behavior Analysis, 23,* 183-195.

Peck, C. A. (1985). Increasing opportunities for social control by children with autism and severe handicaps: Effects on student behavior and perceived classroom climate. *Journal of The Association for Persons with Severe Handicaps, 10,* 133-193.

Reichle, J., York, J., & Eynon, D. (1989). Influence of indicating preferences for initiating, maintaining, and terminating interactions. In F. Brown & D. H. Lehr (Eds.), *Persons with profound disabilities: Issues and practices* (pp. 191-211). Baltimore: Paul H. Brookes.

Shevin, M., & Klein, N. (1984). The importance of choice making skills for students with severe disabilities. *Journal of The Association for Persons with Severe Handicaps, 9,* 159-166.

Sigafoos, J., & Dempsey, R. (1992). Assessing choice making among children with multiple disabilities. *Journal of Applied Behavior Analysis, 25,* 747-755.

Sigafoos, J., Roberts, D., Couzens, D., & Kerr, M. (1993). Providing opportunities for choice-making and turn-taking to adults with multiple disabilities. *Journal of Developmental and Physical Disabilities, 5,* 297-310.